The Holistic Approach to PCOS:

A Complete Guide to Managing Symptoms and Restoring Hormonal Balance

By

Lynda G. Burnley

Preface

Polycystic Ovary Syndrome (PCOS) is a complex and often misunderstood condition that affects millions of women worldwide. While the medical community has made great strides in understanding the underlying hormonal imbalances that contribute to PCOS, many women continue to struggle with managing the symptoms of the condition.

This book provides the latest research on PCOS and the holistic approaches that are effective in managing symptoms and restoring hormonal balance. In this book, you will be provided with a comprehensive guide to the holistic approach to PCOS. Through research and analysis, a wide range of natural and holistic therapies that can help women with PCOS achieve hormonal balance and manage the symptoms of the condition have been identified.

The knowledge in this book will provide a valuable resource for women with PCOS, their families, and healthcare providers, and help to raise awareness of the holistic approach to PCOS. I believe that by working together and adopting a holistic approach, we can improve the lives of millions of women around the world who are affected by this condition.

Table of Contents

Introduction

Polycystic ovary syndrome (PCOS) is a common hormonal disorder that affects women of reproductive age. It can lead to a range of symptoms, including irregular periods, acne, excessive hair growth, and weight gain. In some cases, PCOS can also affect fertility and increase the risk of developing other health conditions, such as type 2 diabetes and heart disease.

The Holistic Approach to PCOS: A Complete Guide to Managing Symptoms and Restoring Hormonal Balance is a comprehensive resource for women with PCOS who are looking for effective and natural ways to manage their symptoms and improve their overall health. This book offers a holistic approach to PCOS management, which means taking into account the whole person - body, mind, and spirit - and addressing the root causes of the condition rather than just treating the symptoms.

Chapter 1 begins by providing an overview of PCOS, including its common symptoms, causes, and risk factors. We also cover how PCOS is diagnosed and what to expect during the diagnostic process.

Chapter 2 focuses on the holistic approach to managing PCOS symptoms. We explained what a holistic approach is and how it can benefit women with PCOS. We also cover various holistic therapies that can help manage PCOS symptoms, including mind-body techniques such as meditation and yoga.

Chapter 3 delves into the role of nutrition and lifestyle changes in managing PCOS. We discussed the best foods to eat and avoid for women with PCOS, as well as the importance of exercise and other lifestyle changes that can help manage symptoms.

Chapter 4 explores alternative and complementary medicine approaches to PCOS management, including herbal medicine, acupuncture, and chiropractic care.

Finally, Chapter 5 addresses PCOS and fertility. We explain how PCOS can affect fertility, the causes and treatments of PCOS-related infertility, and how managing PCOS can improve fertility outcomes. We also cover the risks and management of PCOS during pregnancy.

Whether you've recently been diagnosed with PCOS or have been living with it for years, this book will provide you with a wealth of information and practical tips to help you manage your symptoms and improve your overall health and well-being.

Chapter 1

Understanding Polycystic Ovary Syndrome (PCOS)

Polycystic Ovary Syndrome (PCOS) is a hormonal disorder that affects women of reproductive age. It is a complex condition that can cause a variety of symptoms, including irregular periods, acne, excessive hair growth, and weight gain. While the exact cause of PCOS is not yet fully understood, it is believed to be related to insulin resistance, which can cause hormonal imbalances.

In this chapter, we will discuss the common symptoms, causes, and risk factors of PCOS, as well as the methods used for diagnosing the condition.

1.1 **What is PCOS?**

PCOS is a hormonal disorder that affects the ovaries, which are the female reproductive organs responsible for producing and releasing eggs. Women with PCOS typically have enlarged ovaries that contain small, fluid-filled sacs called cysts. These cysts can cause the ovaries to produce more androgens (male hormones) than normal, which can lead to hormonal imbalances and a range of symptoms.

1.2 Common Symptoms of PCOS

The symptoms of PCOS can vary from woman to woman, and some

women may experience more severe symptoms than others. Some of the most common symptoms of PCOS include:

- Irregular periods or no periods at all
- Excessive hair growth on the face, chest, back, or other parts of the body (known as hirsutism)
- Acne or oily skin
- Weight gain or difficulty losing weight

- Difficulty getting pregnant

- Thinning hair or hair loss

- Darkening of the skin, especially around the neck, groin, and under the breasts

- Sleep apnea

- Mood changes, such as depression or anxiety

1.3 Causes and Risk Factors of PCOS

The exact cause of PCOS is not yet fully understood, but research suggests that it may be related to insulin resistance. Insulin is a hormone that regulates blood sugar levels in the body, and when the body becomes resistant to insulin, it can cause hormonal imbalances and lead to the development of PCOS. Several risk factors can increase a woman's likelihood of developing PCOS, including:

- Family history of PCOS
- Insulin resistance or Type 2 diabetes
- Obesity or overweight

- Sedentary lifestyle

- Unhealthy diet

1.4 **Diagnosing PCOS**

Diagnosing PCOS can be challenging because there is no single test that can definitively diagnose the condition. Instead, doctors typically use a combination of medical history, physical exam, and laboratory tests to make a diagnosis.

To diagnose PCOS, doctors will typically ask about a woman's symptoms and medical history, perform a physical exam, and order blood tests to check hormone levels. Doctors may also perform an ultrasound to look for cysts on the ovaries.

PCOS is a complex condition that can cause a range of symptoms, including irregular periods, excessive hair growth, and weight gain. While the exact cause of PCOS is not yet fully understood, it is believed to be related to insulin resistance. Diagnosing PCOS can be challenging, but a combination of medical history, physical exam, and laboratory tests can help doctors make an accurate diagnosis. In the following chapters, we will discuss various holistic and alternative approaches to managing PCOS symptoms and restoring hormonal balance.

Chapter 2

The Holistic Approach to Managing PCOS Symptoms

Polycystic Ovary Syndrome (PCOS) affects millions of women worldwide, and its symptoms can be both frustrating and overwhelming. The traditional approach to managing PCOS symptoms is often focused solely on medication or surgery. However, a growing number of women are turning to a holistic approach to PCOS management, which considers the whole person, including mind, body, and spirit. In this chapter, we will explore the holistic approach to managing PCOS symptoms, including the benefits of this approach, holistic therapies, and mind-body techniques.

2.1 What is a Holistic Approach?

A holistic approach to health and wellness considers the whole person, including physical, emotional, and spiritual aspects.

Rather than focusing solely on symptoms, a holistic approach seeks to address the underlying causes of health problems. This approach recognizes that the body is an interconnected system and that one area's imbalances can affect others.

For PCOS management, a holistic approach considers factors such as diet, exercise, stress levels, sleep habits, and emotional well-being. It recognizes that PCOS is not just a hormonal condition but a complex interplay of genetic, environmental, and lifestyle factors.

2.2 Benefits of a Holistic Approach to PCOS Management

There are many benefits to taking a holistic approach to PCOS management. One of the most significant benefits is that it empowers women to take an active role in their health and well-being. Rather than feeling like victims of their condition, women can take control of their health by making positive changes in their lifestyle and mindset.

A holistic approach can also help women manage PCOS symptoms more effectively. For example, dietary changes, such as reducing sugar and refined carbohydrates, can help regulate insulin levels and reduce the severity of symptoms such as acne and hair loss. Exercise can help improve insulin sensitivity, boost energy levels, and reduce stress. Mind-body techniques such as meditation, yoga, and deep breathing can help reduce stress and improve emotional well-being, which can have a positive impact on hormone levels.

In addition to managing PCOS symptoms, a holistic approach can improve overall health and well-being. For example, a healthy diet and regular exercise can help prevent conditions such as diabetes and heart disease, which are more common in women with PCOS.

2.3 Holistic Therapies for PCOS Symptoms Management

Many holistic therapies can help manage PCOS symptoms. Here are a few examples:

- Acupuncture: This ancient Chinese therapy involves the insertion of thin needles into specific points on the body. Acupuncture has been shown to help regulate menstrual cycles, reduce insulin resistance, and improve fertility in women with PCOS.

- Herbal medicine: Certain herbs such as saw palmetto, liquorice root, and chaste berry have been shown to help regulate hormones and improve PCOS symptoms.

- Massage therapy: Massage can help reduce stress, improve circulation, and reduce pain and tension in the body.

- Nutritional therapy: Working with a nutritionist can help women with PCOS develop a healthy eating plan that supports hormone balance and reduces inflammation.

2.4 Mind-Body Techniques for PCOS Symptoms Management

In addition to holistic therapies, many mind-body techniques can help manage PCOS symptoms. Here are a few examples:

- Meditation: Meditation involves quieting the mind and focusing on the present moment. It has been shown to reduce stress, improve emotional well-being, and regulate hormone levels.

- Yoga: Yoga combines physical postures with deep breathing and relaxation techniques. It can help reduce stress, improve flexibility, and regulate hormone levels.

- Deep breathing: Deep breathing exercises can help reduce stress and improve relaxation.

- Mindfulness: Mindfulness involves paying attention to the present moment without judgment. It can help reduce stress and improve emotional well-being.

Chapter 3

Nutrition and Lifestyle Changes for PCOS Management

Polycystic ovary syndrome (PCOS) is a hormonal disorder that affects women of reproductive age. It is characterized by multiple cysts on the ovaries, insulin resistance, and hormonal imbalances that can lead to irregular periods, infertility, acne, and weight gain. While there is no cure for PCOS, it can be managed with nutrition and lifestyle changes that support hormonal balance and insulin sensitivity.

3.1 The Role of Nutrition in Managing PCOS

Nutrition plays a crucial role in PCOS management. The right diet can help manage insulin resistance, lower inflammation, and support hormonal balance. Women with PCOS should aim to eat a balanced diet that includes a variety of nutrient-dense foods.

3.2 Best Foods to Eat and Foods to Avoid with PCOS

Some of the best foods for PCOS management include:

- Complex carbohydrates: Whole grains, legumes, fruits, and vegetables provide fibre and slow-digesting carbs that can help manage blood sugar levels.

- Lean proteins: Fish, chicken, turkey, and legumes are

excellent sources of protein
that can help stabilize blood
sugar levels and support
hormone balance.

- Healthy fats: Olive oil,
avocado, nuts, and seeds
provide healthy fats that
support hormone balance and
reduce inflammation.

- Foods rich in antioxidants:
Berries, dark chocolate, and
green leafy vegetables are rich

in antioxidants that can help reduce inflammation and improve insulin sensitivity. On the other hand, it is advisable to avoid or limit certain foods that can worsen PCOS symptoms, such as:

- Processed and high-glycemic-index foods: White bread, sugary drinks, and junk food can cause blood sugar spikes and worsen insulin resistance.

- Dairy products: Some studies suggest that dairy products may contribute to hormonal imbalances and inflammation in women with PCOS.

- Red meat: High intake of red meat has been linked to an increased risk of insulin resistance and inflammation in women with PCOS.

3.3 Importance of Exercise in PCOS Management

Exercise is essential for PCOS management. Regular physical activity can improve insulin sensitivity, support weight loss, and reduce inflammation. Women with PCOS should aim to do at least 150 minutes of moderate-intensity aerobic exercise per week, such as brisk walking, cycling, or swimming. Strength training can also help build muscle mass and improve insulin sensitivity.

3.4 Other Lifestyle Changes for PCOS Management

In addition to nutrition and exercise, other lifestyle changes can help manage PCOS symptoms, including:

- Stress management: Chronic stress can worsen PCOS symptoms by increasing inflammation and insulin resistance. Women with PCOS should aim to manage stress through practices such as yoga,

meditation, or deep breathing
exercises.

- Sleep hygiene: Poor sleep
quality can worsen insulin
resistance and hormonal
imbalances. Women with
PCOS should aim to get at
least 7-8 hours of restful sleep
per night.

- Quit smoking: Smoking has
been linked to increased
inflammation and insulin

resistance in women with PCOS. Quitting smoking can improve overall health and reduce PCOS symptoms.

Managing PCOS through nutrition and lifestyle changes can be challenging, but with a compassionate approach, it is possible to achieve long-term success. Women with PCOS should aim to make sustainable changes that support hormonal balance and overall health, rather than focusing on restrictive diets or excessive exercise regimes. Consultation with a registered dietitian or a healthcare professional can help develop a personalised PCOS management plan.

Chapter 4

Alternative and Complementary Medicine for PCOS Management

Polycystic ovary syndrome (PCOS) is a complex endocrine disorder affecting women of reproductive age. While conventional treatments for PCOS include lifestyle modifications, hormonal therapy, and surgery, some women turn to alternative and complementary medicine approaches for managing their symptoms. This chapter explores some of the most common alternative medicine approaches for PCOS, including herbal medicine, acupuncture, chiropractic care, and other alternative medicine therapies.

4.1 Herbal Medicine for PCOS

Herbal medicine has been used for centuries to treat a variety of health conditions, including PCOS. Some herbs that are commonly used to manage PCOS symptoms include:

- Cinnamon: Cinnamon is
  believed to help regulate
  insulin levels, which can be
  beneficial for women with
  PCOS who are insulin
  resistant. Some studies have
  shown that taking cinnamon
  supplements can help reduce
  insulin resistance and improve
  menstrual cycles in women
  with PCOS.

- Saw palmetto: Saw palmetto is
  a palm tree commonly used to

treat hair loss and acne in women with PCOS. Saw palmetto is believed to reduce the levels of androgen hormones in the body, which can improve symptoms of PCOS.

- Licorice root: Licorice root has been used in traditional medicine to treat a variety of health conditions, including PCOS. Licorice root is believed to help regulate hormone levels in women with PCOS and may also help reduce inflammation in the body.

While some herbs may be beneficial for managing PCOS symptoms, it's important to speak with a healthcare provider before taking any herbal supplements. Some herbs may interact with medications or have side effects.

4.2 Acupuncture for PCOS Management

Acupuncture is a traditional Chinese medicine practice that involves inserting thin needles into specific points on the body. Acupuncture is effective for managing a variety of health conditions, including PCOS. Some studies have shown that acupuncture can help regulate menstrual cycles, reduce insulin resistance, and improve fertility in women with PCOS.

Acupuncture is generally considered safe when performed by a licensed practitioner. However, some women may experience mild side effects, such as soreness, bruising, or dizziness, after an acupuncture session.

4.3 Chiropractic Care for PCOS Management

Chiropractic care is a form of alternative medicine that focuses on the musculoskeletal system. While chiropractic care is not typically used to treat PCOS directly, some women with PCOS may benefit from chiropractic adjustments to relieve back pain, neck pain, and other musculoskeletal symptoms. Chiropractic care is generally considered safe when performed by a licensed chiropractor. However, some women with PCOS may need to avoid certain chiropractic techniques that involve the lower back or abdomen, as these areas can be sensitive in women with PCOS

4.4 Other Alternative Medicine Approaches for PCOS

In addition to herbal medicine, acupuncture, and chiropractic care, several other alternative medicine approaches may be beneficial for managing PCOS symptoms, including;

Mind-body therapies, such as yoga, meditation, and mindfulness, which may help reduce stress and improve overall well-being in women with PCOS.

Dietary supplements, such as omega-3 fatty acids, vitamin D, and inositol, may help improve insulin resistance and other PCOS symptoms.

Traditional Chinese medicine, such as herbal remedies and acupuncture, may help regulate menstrual cycles and reduce PCOS symptoms.

While alternative medicine approaches may be beneficial for managing PCOS symptoms, it's important to remember that they are not a substitute for conventional medical treatments. Women with PCOS should work closely with their healthcare providers to develop a comprehensive treatment plan that includes both conventional and alternative medicine approaches.

Chapter 5

PCOS and Fertility

5.1 Understanding PCOS and Fertility

Polycystic Ovary Syndrome (PCOS) is a hormonal disorder that affects women of reproductive age. Women with PCOS experience a range of symptoms, including irregular periods, excess facial and body hair, acne, weight gain, and infertility. One of the main challenges faced by women with PCOS is difficulty getting pregnant, due to irregular ovulation and hormonal imbalances.

PCOS affects the functioning of the ovaries, which may result in the development of small cysts on the ovaries. These cysts can affect the production and release of hormones, such as estrogen, progesterone, and testosterone, which are important for ovulation and fertility. The exact cause of PCOS is not yet fully understood, but researchers believe it is related to genetics, insulin resistance, and inflammation.

5.2 PCOS and Infertility: Causes and Treatments

Infertility is a common complication of PCOS, affecting up to 80% of women with the condition. Irregular ovulation and hormonal imbalances can make it difficult for women with PCOS to get pregnant naturally. In some cases, women with PCOS may require medical intervention to achieve pregnancy.

There are several treatment options available for infertility caused by PCOS. These include lifestyle changes, such as losing weight and managing insulin resistance through diet and exercise. Women with PCOS may also benefit from medications to stimulate ovulation, such as clomiphene citrate or letrozole. In some cases, assisted reproductive technologies (ART) such as in vitro fertilization (IVF) may be necessary.

5.3 Managing PCOS to Improve Fertility

Managing PCOS can help improve fertility outcomes for women with the condition. Lifestyle changes, such as maintaining a healthy weight, eating a balanced diet, and engaging in regular exercise, can help manage insulin resistance and improve ovulation. Medications, such as metformin, may also help manage insulin resistance and improve ovulation.

In addition to managing insulin resistance, managing other symptoms of PCOS, such as acne and excess hair growth, can also improve fertility outcomes. Hormonal birth control may be prescribed to regulate periods and reduce the risk of developing ovarian cysts.

5.4 PCOS and Pregnancy: Risks and Management

Women with PCOS are at higher risk of complications during pregnancy, including gestational diabetes, preeclampsia, and preterm delivery. However, with proper management and monitoring, most women with PCOS can have a healthy pregnancy and delivery. Women with PCOS who are planning to become pregnant should work closely with their healthcare providers to manage their condition and reduce the risk of complications. This may include regular monitoring of blood sugar levels, blood pressure, and fetal development. Medications used to manage PCOS may need to be adjusted or discontinued during pregnancy, so it is important to consult with a healthcare provider before starting or stopping any medications.

PCOS is a hormonal disorder that can affect fertility in women. However, with proper management and treatment, most women with PCOS can achieve pregnancy and have a healthy baby. Managing insulin resistance through lifestyle changes and medication, and monitoring for complications during pregnancy, are key components of managing PCOS and improving fertility outcomes.

Conclusion

Polycystic Ovary Syndrome (PCOS) is a complex condition that affects millions of women worldwide. While there is no cure for PCOS, there are a range of treatments available that can help manage symptoms and improve quality of life. However, many of these treatments involve the use of medications that can have unpleasant side effects or invasive procedures such as surgery.

In recent years, there has been growing interest in the use of natural and holistic therapies to manage PCOS symptoms and restore hormonal balance. Through my research and analysis, I have identified a range of natural and holistic therapies that can help women with PCOS to achieve hormonal balance and manage the symptoms of the condition.

These therapies include dietary changes, exercise, stress reduction techniques, and natural supplements. By adopting a holistic approach to PCOS, women can take control of their health and well-being, and reduce the impact of the condition on their lives.

I believe that the holistic approach to PCOS offers a promising alternative to traditional medical treatments, and has the potential to improve the lives of millions of women around the world who are affected by this condition.

In writing this book, I have aimed to provide a comprehensive guide to the holistic approach to PCOS, based on the latest research and scientific evidence. I hope that this book will serve as a valuable resource for women with PCOS, their families, and healthcare providers, and help to raise awareness of the holistic approach to PCOS.

I encourage all women with PCOS to explore the natural and holistic therapies discussed in this book and to work with their healthcare providers to develop a personalized treatment plan that meets their individual needs. With the right tools and support, women with PCOS can achieve hormonal balance and lead happy, healthy lives.